DIÓMEDES BAIGORRIA

DENTAL MALPRACTICE

DIÓMEDES BAIGORRIA

DENTAL MALPRACTICE

A CONTEMPORARY LEGAL VIEW

ScienciaScripts

Imprint

Any brand names and product names mentioned in this book are subject to trademark, brand or patent protection and are trademarks or registered trademarks of their respective holders. The use of brand names, product names, common names, trade names, product descriptions etc. even without a particular marking in this work is in no way to be construed to mean that such names may be regarded as unrestricted in respect of trademark and brand protection legislation and could thus be used by anyone.

Cover image: www.ingimage.com

This book is a translation from the original published under ISBN 978-620-3-87863-9.

Publisher:
Sciencia Scripts
is a trademark of
Dodo Books Indian Ocean Ltd., member of the OmniScriptum S.R.L Publishing group
str. A.Russo 15, of. 61, Chisinau-2068, Republic of Moldova Europe
Printed at: see last page
ISBN: 978-620-4-12906-8

SUMMARY

The object of this monograph is to study the consequences and effects of dental malpractice by the dental professional in the act of caring for a patient, whether in private or public consultation. From a contemporary legal perspective.

The main objective is to promote awareness of the oral health professional, as an act of protocol. Preventive to avoid legal consequences either civil or criminal. By an erroneous practice in the exercise of their profession, this erroneous practice can occur either: by non-observance of protocol procedures or legal regulations, by inexperience, inexperience, or lack of skill (vocation).

Analyzing what is established in the second article of the code of dental ethics, it mentions that the professional performance of the dentist should be adjusted to the following norms:

a) RESPECT FOR LIFE
b) RESPECT FOR THE HUMAN PERSONALITY
c) A SINCERE RECOGNITION OF ONE'S OWN LIMITATIONS.

Malpractice or wrongful practice occurs when it causes damage to the body or health of the person, whether this damage is partial or total, limited in time or permanent as a result of a professional action performed with recklessness or negligence, or lack of expertise in their profession or art of healing, or by failure to comply with the regulations or duties in charge with a departure from the applicable legal standards.

As we can see, this issue of professional practice in dentistry is quite broad and complex.

It is for this reason that in this work we will focus on the analysis of dental malpractice with a contemporary legal version from the point of view of legal documents such as the clinical history of the pathological condition of the patient and the informed and signed consent of the patient to be treated.

Based on the second principle of the standard of care or Lex Artis ADHOC

The law of the art to study it says Morales starts from the following:

- EACH CLINICAL PICTURE GENERATES A DIAGNOSIS
- EVERY DIAGNOSIS GENERATES A BEHAVIOR
- AND ANY BEHAVIOR OR TREATMENT MUST BE

DEFINED:

      . What to do

      . Who should do

      . How to do it

      . When to do

      . For what should be done

KEYWORDS:

Dental Malpractice, Oral Health, Iatrogenesis, Professional Practice, Medical Liability.

Table of Contents

SUMMARY 1

1. - INTRODUCTION 4

2. - PROBLEM STATEMENT.. 5

3. - FORMULATION OF THE PROBLEM 5

4. - OBJECTIVES 5

5. - JUSTIFICATION 6

6. METHODOLOGICAL DESIGN OF THE RESEARCH............................. 7

CHAPTER I 9

PRELIMINARY PART AND MALPRACTICE

IN MEDICAL SCIENCE AND DENTISTRY 9

CHAPTER II 20

THE CIVIL RESPONSIBILITY OF THE DENTIST AND VALUATION

OF THE ELEMENTS OF CIVIL LIABILITY 20

CONCLUSIONS 49

RECOMMENDATIONS 50

INFORMED AND SIGNED CONSENT.. 53

OTHER DOCUMENTS.. 54

PROPOSAL... 55

BIBLIOGRAPHY.. 56

WEBGRAPHY 58

1.   - INTRODUCTION

Malpractice in dentistry is the adverse outcome occurring during a dental act and resulting from an action or omission of the practitioner. It is the proper non-compliance with established rules, principles or precepts.

This adverse outcome occurs during a dental act and caused by some element of fault or incompetence of the dental professional where the patient suffered harm, due to a cause attributable to the performance of the professional who deviated from good practice, or did not respect the rules in force. It is a breach of the rules.

Campos indicates: "The **juridical criterion** that characterizes the professional malpractice of the dentist has to be better defined, where the attention is especially directed to the "Animus" the **intention** of the professional when promoting his work, the **Modus Operandi** that is to say, the **Professional Quality** or, his condition of "Pudens" that is to say, to prudently **respect** the limits imposed by science; to his constant "Cura e Vigilantia" in the **treatment** and its **results**, immediate and mediate. Thus, a dental fact will be transformed into malpractice as soon as it is unequivocally proven that the dentist acted with imperfection or negligence, that is, with at least one of the three behaviors that identify guilt".

In this work we use the qualitative type of research to establish the behavior of the dental professional in the act of professional-patient care that according to its immediate or mediate results can be qualified as right or wrong.

The content of this research paper is organized in three parts:

A first chapter which is preliminary and establishes the criteria of the research profile, concepts and scientific technical terms, in relation to medical-dental malpractice.

A second chapter that describes an analysis from a contemporary legal perspective, in the medical-dental malpractice.

A third chapter that sets out the Conclusions, recommendations and the Proposal.

2.   - PROBLEM STATEMENT

In contemporary dentistry in our plurinational state of Bolivia, taking into account the last decade, it has been observed through the media and social networks, publications of cases of complaints on the subject of medical and dental malpractice, motivated by this situation we decided to address this issue in this paper, in order to identify the origin of the problem, its punitive, civil and / or criminal consequences, in order to provide suggestions and recommendations to contribute to the prevention of these conflicts in the exercise of the medical-dental profession.

3. - PROBLEM FORMULATION

It is necessary to establish a contemporary legal vision of the origin of dental malpractice in contemporary dentistry, perceptible in the society of the Plurinational State of Bolivia?

4. - OBJECTIVES

4.1. - OVERALL OBJECTIVE

Establish and identify the responsibility of the dentist in the act of patient care in the exercise of their oral health treatment and conduct or attitude in the art of healing in the exercise of their profession, from a contemporary legal vision.

4.2. - SPECIFIC OBJECTIVES

1. Identify the legal causes and effects of malpractice in dentistry. Contemporary
2. Identify the valuation of the elements of civil liability.

3. To establish contemporary legal guidelines in relation to the civil liability of the dentist in dental malpractice.

5.   - JUSTIFICATION

The relevant importance of addressing the issue of dental malpractice is based on the reality of contemporary dentistry, due to a growing population explosion of the population that demands the attention of odontostomatologic treatment services, and on the other hand the overpopulation of dental professionals, and the growing creation of faculties and careers of dentistry that sometimes these academic institutions do not fully comply with the plans and programs of studies in their curricular plan in which the subject of legal and forensic dentistry should be inserted and emphasized in order to prevent malpractice of the new professional in society.

That is, the implementation of pedagogical and academic curricular policies for the education and training of new professionals in oral health, and thus ensure the training of professionals to serve our society with efficiency, quality and warmth, duly motivated with a high level vocation and human quality.

The lack of state policy through the governing body such as the Ministry of Education.

And the Ministry of Health. For vocational selection and admission, as well as state policies for the authorization of the ministerial resolution for the opening of academic institutions, universities with faculties and careers in dentistry.

The motivation to approach the present work is also based on the principles of the Political Constitution of the State that in its Art. 8 paragraph 1 and 2 of living well (ama qamaña).

6. METHODOLOGICAL DESIGN OF THE RESEARCH

The research design includes the type of research, methods, techniques and instruments.

6.1. TYPE OF RESEARCH

6.1.1. Type of research qualitative

Qualitative research is about discovering knowledge without numerical measurement, where variables are described through case study research. The researcher asks general and open-ended questions, collects data expressed through written, verbal and non-verbal language, as well as visual, which he describes and analyzes and turns into themes. Qualitative research is based on a perspective focused on understanding the meaning of the actions of living beings, mainly humans and their institutions.

6.1.2. Type of research descriptive

It is descriptive in that it describes the concepts, characteristics and details in relation to dental malpractice.

6.2. METHODS

The methods will be interpretative, analytical and comparative.

6.2.1 Legal Interpretive Method

The legal interpretative method will be used to analyze the Bolivian legal regulations, to assign its scope, and its form will be systemic, since it is necessary to establish the right to health, life and physical integrity of persons.

6.2.2. Analytical method

A breakdown of the integral parts of dental malpractice will be made, such as its procedures, rights, criminal liability and the reparation of material, corporal and moral damages caused by this crime.

7

6.2.3. Deductive Method - The deductive method operates from general characterizations to arrive at particularities and specificities in research, e.g., from general medicine to dental practice.

6.3. TECHNIQUES

The technique will be documentary or bibliographic.

6.3.1. Documentary technique

To approach the systematic and structured research of a particular study it is necessary to have a theoretical support, which derives from the review of documents, Books, Articles, Texts, Reports, which have bibliographic reproduction either in a traditional or computerized context with the help of the internet.

6.4. INSTRUMENTS

The data collection instruments are bibliographic cards.

6.4.1. Textual bibliographic sheets

The textual bibliographic cards will be used to extract from the legal and doctrinal sources the necessary citations for the processing of theoretical information.

CHAPTER I

PRELIMINARY PART AND MALPRACTICE

IN MEDICAL SCIENCE AND DENTISTRY

1.1. - PRELIMINARY PART

Today as yesterday and in front of the cases that are denounced by the different media, it is necessary to remember what "medical responsibility" implies, understanding that this is the set of actions that the legal and normative system imposes on the physician, constituting an obligation to respond for the consequences that may cause damage in our professional activity.

History allows us to recall premises, principles and cases that have established current jurisprudence, for example:

The Code of Hammurabi that established the death penalty or the amputation of the hands to the doctor who did not attend with prudence and with the necessary care.

Hippocrates, who established the ethical standards of the time by means of rational and natural principles and bases in Greek medicine.

Remember that in the times of the Roman Empire imperfection was punished with a pecuniary sanction.

The cases of Dr. Helie, 1825, which through an opinion of the Academy of Medicine, the court of Dromfont imposes the doctor to pay a "life pension" to the patient concerned. And the case of Dr. Thouret, Noroy 1832, which for negligence and negligence obliges the doctor to compensate the damage through an "indemnity".

Therefore, the medical act involves 2 types of liability:

Criminal Liability, which constitutes a social harm and a crime.

And Civil Liability. The latter, as it constitutes a particular damage, requires the reparation of the same.

When the doctor is sued in the ordinary way, most of the acts that cause harm to the patient are of "Culpable" nature (without the intention of producing it), describing 4 forms that are sometimes confused, so it is necessary to remember them:

The Impericia. It is the lack of minimum or basic knowledge necessary for the correct performance of the medical act. It is the "inexcusable ignorance" or the performance of the professional with technical ineptitude, this may result from the lack of regular updating of the practitioner.

Negligence. Which is the act of the professional with "carelessness and inattention". It therefore constitutes the "inexcusable omission".

Recklessness. The doctor acting with excessive confidence. It is the "inexcusable recklessness", therefore lack of foresight or caution in the professional act.

Non-compliance with regulations. This occurs when a requirement or rule (verbal or written) is omitted. Unfortunately when the damage has occurred, there are consequences related to criminal liability can mean imprisonment. Therefore acts typifiable as a crime. Civil liability in most cases requires a pecuniary (i.e. financial) penalty.

However, when analyzing all the factors involved in the production of patient harm, there are clearly three distinguishable levels:

On the part of the doctor:

The physician's actions must be based on scientific solvency, moral integrity, objectivity, impartiality, humility and methodology.

On the part of the patient:

Compliance with the therapeutic plan, loyalty to the physician and good faith are required.

On the part of the intermediate bodies (managing bodies):

The provision of adequate systems of assistance, care, monitoring and control.

The existence of supplies, medicines and equipment that guarantee good medical practice.

The staff, which must be sufficient and with the required technical capacity.

In addition to the aforementioned, 2 problems have also been observed that constitute aggravating factors at the time of a judicial defense: the illegal exercise of the profession and the medical specialty.

In relation to the illegal practice of the profession, this occurs when the alleged practitioner is not really a doctor.

In relation to the illegal exercise of the specialty, it is established when:

The specialist does not demonstrate to have been trained in the minimum time of formation that the norm establishes it and under the System of Medical Residence, as the only system recognized by the national norm as well as international.

In cases where specialist certificates were granted only for years of seniority, without taking into account the criteria or national regulations established by the corresponding Scientific Society and the Medical College, since there is really no necessary education and training, constituting in reality a form of empiricism.

When the years of training have been reduced due to the premise of insufficient specialized human resources, this generates professionals with poor resolution capacity and inadequate technical training.

And if the Specialist Certification and/or the University degree have not taken into account the criteria of the particular Scientific Society registered in the table of years of training and recognized in the Statutes and Regulations of the Medical College of Bolivia.

In summary, there is enough normative and legal body that is brought up as a basis for the analysis of this editorial, to cite:

Law 3131, art 4, art 6, art 7, art 11, art 12, art 13, art 14, art 18.

Regulation of Medical Specialties and Subspecialties of the Organic Statute and Regulations of the Medical College of Bolivia.

Penal Code of Bolivia, art 260, art 263 to art 269, art 270, art 271 to art 274.

Bolivian Civil Code, art 6, art 18, art 984.

New Political Constitution of the Plurinational State of Bolivia. Art. 9, inc 5, art 18, art 35 to 45, art 321.

The medical responsibility begins and ends respecting the current regulations, having as a premise the benefit of the patient, to whom we owe ourselves.

1.2. - MALPRACTICE IN MEDICAL SCIENCE - DENTISTRY

In the field of Deontology and in a very general way, Morales Martínez, proposes principles with which we must work: **(MORALES MARTÍNEZ, PEDRO. "El patólogo en la investigación por responsabilidad medica" Revista del Instituto Nacional de Medicina Legal de Colombia. Volume XVI 2016.**

- Principle of Duty,
- Standard of Care Principle,
- Principle of Harm

1.2.1. - PRINCIPLE OF DUTY

It refers to the duty or obligation of the professional to provide care to a patient, establishing the dentist-patient relationship, which is generated when the patient comes to the consultation, whether private or public. The violation of this principle occurs when the dentist accepts the patient's care, but does not comply with it.

1.2.2. - PRINCIPLE OF THE STANDARD OF CARE OR LEX ARTIS AD HOC

The Law of Art. To study it, says Morales, we start from the following:

Each clinical picture generates a diagnosis

Every diagnosis generates a behavior

In all conduct or treatment must be defined: what should be done, who should do it, how it should be done, when it should be done, why it should be done When analyzing the standard of care, it must be established if according to the signs and symptoms presented by the patient, a diagnosis was established rationally made, if he was given adequate and timely treatment, for this purpose several factors are taken into account:

- Technical and scientific resources

- Human resources
- Financial and administrative resources

Taking into account that the limitations should **not** be of knowledge, skills or abilities.

Lex Artis, then, is the **application of the general rules of dentistry to the same or similar cases.** It is the way we proceed for the same fact or disease.

A modern concept, it refers to the "exercise with probability results" but requires "mastering the subjects of the profession" (Ocampo) to have a probable outcome.

The Lex Artis, has **conditions,** where the constant evolution with science is demanded (Century of Surgery), because we are in the base of the "Culture of Health".

Also, it has elements:

- **Professional suitability,** which is a specific quality to exercise this profession.

- **Study and analysis prior** to the odontological act. **(MORALES MARTÍNEZ, PEDRO. "The pathologist in the investigation by responsibility.**

  medica" Journal of the National Institute of Legal Medicine of Colombia. Volume XVI. Page 78 2016).

Dedication to the profession, and to the patient, giving him/her the necessary time to explain his/her problem and to understand our explanation when asking for consent, time for the evaluation of the complementary tests, time for the diagnosis and for the treatment.

The Lex Artis, has **indications:**

- Evaluates the Risk-Benefit binomial
- Treatment indicated to the specific case.
- Avoid obsolete techniques and materials.

Lex Artis has **requirements:**

- That the correct technique has been applied, at the correct age, with the correct material.
  - Respect for essential principles.
  - Adherence to Deontological standards.

The Lex Artis has **objectives:**

- Find or rule out the causal element.
- Demarcate the result obtained.
- Demonstrate the circumstances that led to the event.

The Code of Dental Ethics mentions that the professional performance of the dentist must be fundamentally adjusted to the following norms (Art. 2):

a) Respect for life.

b) I respect human personality.

c) Sincere recognition of one's own limitations.

It should also be projected with the community, with colleagues, etc. (Art. 3 °).

There is a distortion of the concept of ethics when the Professional Fees are incompatible with the economic situation of a region or a sector, or when we are aware of the idiosyncrasy of the population (middle or low strata), and we do not provide them with a third or fourth level care, in a particular way.

1.2.3. - PRINCIPLE OF HARM

"Non daeneare", thou shalt not harm, "no one is allowed to cause harm to another..." (Page 33)

1.2.4. - HEALTH MALPRACTICE

lraola explains that malpractice or malpractice occurs when damage is caused to the body or health of the person, whether this damage is partial or total, limited in time or permanent, as a consequence of a professional action carried out with imprudence or negligence, lack of skill in their profession or art of healing or by non-observance of the regulations or duties in their charge with deviation from the applicable legal regulations. **(IRAOLA, Lidia. Medical-legal liability and malpractice. Lp. 2014).**

It is harmful or harmful to health when the foreseeable damage was not foreseen, or trusted that it could avoid it, without achieving it. It can be an inconstant damage, avoidable with a good professional practice, there must be a causal relationship, with a variable time of occurrence, and sometimes caused by professional incompetence.

1.2.5. - MALPRACTICE IN DENTISTRY

It is the adverse outcome occurring during a dental act and resulting from an action or omission of the professional. It is the proper non-compliance with established rules, principles or precepts. This adverse result occurs during a dental act and caused by some element of fault, or incompetence, etc. of the dental professional where the patient suffered damage due to a cause attributable to the performance of the professional, who deviated from good practice or did not respect the rules in force. It is the "breaking of the rules".

Campos indicates that "the **juridical criterion** that characterizes the professional malpractice of the dentist has to be better defined, where the attention is directed, specifically, to the "animus", the **intention** of the professional when proposing his work; to the "modus operandi", that is the **professional quality;** to his condition of "prudens", that is, to **respect** prudently the limits imposed by science; to his constant "cura et vigilantia", in the **treatment** and its **results,** immediate and mediate. Thus, a dental fact will be transformed into malpractice as soon as it is proven, unequivocally, that the dentist acted with inexperience, imprudence or negligence, that is, with at least one of the three behaviors that identify culpability". (**MORALES MARTÍNEZ, PEDRO. "El patólogo en la investigación por responsabilidad medica" Revista del Instituto Nacional de Medicina Legal de Colombia. Volume XVI. Page 85 2016)**

According to a **dental criterion**, in practice, the facts attributable to malpractice are much broader but less precise. Anything that happens to a patient, due to the action and/or omission of the dentist, would be malpractice.

Many errors are excusable facts, as long as the professional has used, correctly and opportunely, the knowledge and rules of the current dental science, having only had an unforeseeable event. For this reason, many authors do not even consider them professional errors, in the sense of malpractice.

When an adverse event occurs in patients, they come to the College of Dentists asking for an ethical and disciplinary sanction for the professional, or to mediate between the patient and the dentist seeking redress. Therefore, the Colleges should become Courts of Conciliation and Arbitration. And, it is here where dentists should seek to end the conflict and not wait for the problem to reach the judicial spheres.

Examples of malpractice can be when in a root canal treatment there is the ingestion of an instrument into the digestive tract or the fall of foreign bodies through the trachea, the migration of implants, buccosinusal communications, traumatic exodontia, leaving broken needles, fracturing maxillae, producing hematomas by infiltration in canal irrigation, a drop of camphor paramonoclofenol or phosphoric acid in the patient's lips, etc..., everything becomes malpractice; if the operating agent does not immediately solve the damage caused to the patient or refer to a specialist to help him to solve that lack of care.

The most advisable thing to do is to explain to the patient what happened, to show that there was no intention to harm at any time, that all possible resources were used. Be concerned, understand that we are adding to his suffering. Let's not be indolent, and let's not send him home with that problem that we could not solve. How we behave, at that moment, we will have to answer to Justice, since in the complaints for malpractice, which are ventilated in court, the abandonment of the patient, the omission of the duties of care, the arrogance, the inattention shown by the professional, rather than the damage itself, are more important.

Finally, some errors in diagnosis or treatment may be excusable, but they must be proven.

1.2.6. - GENERAL FACTORS THAT DETERMINE MALPRACTICE

Already in 1962, Professor Graga Leite, quoted by Campos, proposed four factors that explained the professional errors:

- Pressure from the economic factor.
- Moral fragility.
- Lack of professional vocation.
- Omission of basic scientific rules

Today, we can add other factors:

- Indiscriminate increase in the number of dental schools, with defects in professional training.

- The massification of teaching; for a profession that is still an art;

18

the collaboration of assistants or professionals, assistants or guests, is essential.

• Lack of good communication with patients.

• Submission to inadequate and/or precarious working conditions.

• Anomie or near certainty of impunity for adverse outcomes.

• Self-confidence in the co-operativeness expected of dental experts and dental associations.

Gisbert Calabuig5 explains that the increase in malpractice suits is due to "the number of professionals, the progress in the treatment of diseases that until recently were incurable, the triumphalism with which the advances of this science are disseminated, which leads to consider the cure as a right, and also to the search for economic benefits through compensation litigation" (Gisbert Calabuig, J.A., "Medicina Legal y la Medicina Legal y la Medicina Legal y la Médecina"). (**GISBERT CALABUIG, J.A., "Legal Medicine and Toxicology", Barcelona, Masson-Salvat, 1992).**

CHAPTER II

THE CIVIL RESPONSIBILITY OF THE DENTIST AND VALUATION

OF THE ELEMENTS OF CIVIL LIABILITY

2.1. - THE CIVIL LIABILITY OF THE DENTIST

2.1.1. - DEFINITIONS

Civil liability is that which arises from the breach of the obligation of contractual or extra-contractual origin.

This liability translates into the need for the professional, with the victim to repair or compensate the damage suffered as a result of his wilful or negligent action or omission. (**COSTA ARDUZ Rolando, COSTA B. Dario. Medical Legal Terms in the Bolivian Legislation. 2005**)

Civil liability of the dentist, when that derives from a dental act, is the obligation to satisfy the effects that derive from faults that cause damage or harm.
(RODRIGUEZ A. Civil Liability Derived from the Medical Act. Colombia. 2004).

It is not that there is a particular or different liability regime for health professionals, with respect to the rest of the subjects of law, but the ways of incurring liability for facts derived from the practice of dentistry are the subject of particular study.

2.1.2. - FUNDAMENTALS
- The expression "pas de responsabilité sans faute", means that "there *is* no *responsibility without fault*".
- It is the basis of tort law.

- It is born from the "Theory of Damage, Fault and the Theory of Causation", and others.

- It has more to do with reparation and prevention than punishment.

- Nowadays, jurisprudence is no longer based on the punishment of the tortfeasor, nor on revenge. Now where the punishment is based, is in the patrimony of the one who has caused the illicit act; trying to return the patient to his original state, to the integrity that he enjoyed before having suffered damage.

- The **preventive** aspect is to ensure that we act prudently, to avoid liability. It is about minimizing the negative influences that the professional's activity may have on others, because when dentists who cause harm assume the costs of the damage they cause, we will have the necessary incentives to take precautionary measures to avoid them.

2.1.3. - CLASSIFICATION OF CIVIL LIABILITY There are many classifications, we will take only the one that interests us: **(VILLARROEL BUSTIOS, CESAR.**
"Obligations" Law School. UMSA. 2005).

By its nature. It is divided into contractual and non-contractual:

2.I.3.I.   - CONTRACTUAL RELATION

Article 450.- (NONNOTION). There is a contract when two or more persons agree to constitute, modify or extinguish a legal relationship between them. CC.

Article 452.- (REQUIREMENTS). For the formation of a contract, it is required:
a) Consent.

21

b) Object.

c) Cause, and

d) **Form, provided it** is legally enforceable. CC

It will be a real contract, when the last clause (Written and signed) has been fulfilled.

The Contract to work in Health or the Assignment of work, guarantees a result, it obliges to fulfill what has been promised. In case of breach, we have to respond according to the degree of responsibility that has been offered (Rehabilitative and Aesthetic Dentistry, Orthodontics).

The **contract of services or service contract,** when the professional has to perform a task for the benefit of the patient, but is not obliged to a result. That is, it is not obliged to cure, but to act with diligence! to improve the current state of the patient, using all the scientific and technological knowledge that is available to them.

CHARACTERISTICS OF A CONTRACT

- Bilateral
- Presumed onerous
- Consensual,
- Successive tract (Permanent or instantaneous)
- It is intuito personae
- Principal (Yungano) .admits the existence of accessory contracts, such as laboratory analyses, Rx, etc.

THE CONTRACTUAL CIVIL LIABILITY, that supposes a pre-existing legal bond; it is the one that comes from the **breach of** a contract and consists of the obligation to compensate the patient for the damage that we caused him/her because we have breached a contract or that there is a late or imperfect breach.

In order for contractual liability to proceed, three requirements must be met:

1. Existence of a contract (Bolivian jurists affirm that it is sufficient that there has been a verbal agreement, a contract has been generated).

2. That one of the parties causes damage to the detriment of the other party. That the damage arises from the non-performance, non-execution or defective execution of the contracted obligation (disobturation, fractures).

2.I.3.2.   - NON-CONTRACTUAL RELATIONSHIP

Established without prior bond, but predetermined, assumed or imposed by law.

THE EXTRACONTRACTUAL CIVIL LIABILITY, is the one that comes from the breach of an obligation where there is no previous existing link between the patient and the author of the damage. Where the patient is deprived of his volitional capacity (will), can not decide, occurs in states of unconsciousness, epileptic seizures, accidents and others and requires urgent attention. The omission, enters the field of Criminal Liability. The Extracontractual Civil Liability is divided into:

a) Legal Liability

b) Civil liability for tort or wrongful act.

a) Legal tort liability,

When the damage originated in an involuntary fault without intention. It is precisely the act committed which gives rise to the obligation to compensate him.

b) Extra-contractual tort liability, called by the Romans Civil offence.

The prefixed conduct, predetermined by law, is not described but assumed, it is a conduct of not causing harm to another.

A sanction is imposed in the case of non-compliance and it is to compensate the damage.

Art. 984 CC (REMEDY FOR UNLAWFUL DEED).

"Whoever, by an intentional or negligent act, causes someone an unjust damage, is obliged to compensate".

REQUIREMENTS FOR TORT LIABILITY.

In order for tort liability to proceed, the following requirements are necessary:

The damage.

Guilt or **malice** is found in Art. 14. "The person who commits an act foreseen in a criminal offence with knowledge and will is guilty of malice. For this it is sufficient that the perpetrator seriously considers possible its realization and accepts this possibility". C.P.

It is also defined as "The consciousness of *wanting* and the consciousness of *acting,* translated into an external conduct, that is to say, it is the conscious will, directed or oriented to the perpetration of an act that the law foresees as a crime".

Therefore, it assumes a preconceived desire to cause harm, whoever acts with malice commits a civil and criminal offence. Whoever alleges malice must prove it, it is not presumed.

Luna distinguishes three meanings: **(LUNA YAÑEZ Alberto. "Obligations". Printing. Artyk productions. 1996).**

Fraud as a vice of the will,
Fraud as an element of wrongful acts,
Fraud in the breach of obligations of conventional origin.

We will relate a case where a colleague acted with malice, "...when the dentist found out that the patient she was attending was her husband's "other" partner, she proposed a series of dental treatments, which according to the professional she needed them in a hurry. The patient agreed, since she did not know that her dentist was the wife of her current partner.

Each dental session was carried out practically without anesthesia, with the excuse that this was the only way to treat this type of problem. He placed arsenic on all the healthy teeth, changing them every other day, causing the patient unbearable pain. He performed unnecessary root canals and extractions. The patient could not stand it any longer and consulted another professional, who informed her of the unnecessary treatments, irreversible damage to the anterior teeth and signs of osteomyelitis in both jaws...". (1985) consequence of the subjective system adopted by our Civil Code. (**DE BRIGARD PEREZ Ana. Fault in medical liability. Colombia).**

Only persons who lack the discernment necessary to be aware of the acts they perform are incapable.

Difference between contractual liability and non-contractual liability.

The **non-contractual liability** known as "aquiliana" must prove the

25

existence of fault on the part of the professional, while in the **contractual** liability it is sufficient to prove the **breach of the** obligation arising from the contract.

On this point, in a Judgment of the Supreme Court of Chile, it mentions "both responsibilities have common presuppositions, especially in the production of **damage** and the **existence of fault.** The **degree** of liability is more in the contractual one". (www.negligenciasmedicas.)

They also vary in the length of time they are **prescribed.**

The **anti-juridical conduct,** originating a damage has different sanctions, whether subjective or objective.

The **capacity** to contract is required in the contractual one, on the other hand the extra-contractual one can be born without it.

All of the above is important to avoid duplication of compensation.

Another Sentence of the same Supreme Court, expresses ".... the creditor (for us the patient), in the contractual relationship, who acts or initiates the process must **prove the obligation** and **characteristics of the provision** (reason for consultation), if it is of means or result - as well as the **non-compliance,** if the professional has not acted under the observance of the duties of that provision, then you can oppose, upon proof, **the payment or its fulfillment.**

On the contrary, in non-contractual liability, the injured party (patient) will have to prove not only the damage, but also the **authorship of the harmful conduct, the causal link and the voluntariness** of the authorship for infringing duties of prevention".

2.1.4. - DENTIST - PATIENT LEGAL RELATIONSHIP

When this relationship is given in the light of an institution where the dentist is dependent on that entity, there will be a contractual relationship of a civil nature, by the fact of his dependent, should be responsible for the entity to which it belongs.

When it is in a decentralized public entity, it is a non-contractual relationship of the State. [10]

In some situations the contractual and non-contractual relationship can exist indistinctly - with the general duty to act with diligence and prudence and not to cause harm to another - e.g. When simple exodontia are complicated (contractual), unforeseen alveolectomies or odontosections can be performed (non-contractual).

When the patient goes to a Health Service, whether public or private, he/she enters into a contract with the Institution, not directly with the professional. And, according to the standards of care of that service, patients are sorted to certain professionals, that is to say, the dentists are imposed on them, they do not choose them.

When a harmful event occurs due to the actions of these professionals, it is the Institution who is responsible for the third parties, since it is the Institution that hires its personnel and, therefore, the Responsibility is of the Institution (Ramello).

Félix Trigo Represas, quoted by **Sabat,** calls this type of liability **"Stipulation in favor of** third parties", where the institution enters into a contract with the professional and the latter is obliged to perform a service, not for the benefit of the institution, but for the benefit of the patient. The patient is the one who enters into a reflex contract with the Institution and a direct contract with the professional. In situations of Professional Responsibility, it is the Health Institution that must respond for the dentist **(SABAT, JOSÉ. "Diplomado de Responsabilidad Civil y Penal de los médicos". Argentine Professor. Law. UMSA.2008**

Alberto Baures, disagrees with Trigo, distinguishing the responsibility of the Health Institution with the patient as direct contractual relations and not reflexes, with the duty of specific fulfillment of the obligation. **(SABAT, JOSÉ. "Diplomado de Responsabilidad Civil y Penal de los médicos". Argentine Teacher. Law. UMSA. 2008)**

Also, because the Institution has the Principle of the Tacit Duty of Security (Tacit, when it is presumed of certain facts or acts) and the Institution is responsible if there is a malpractice on the part of its professional. And, also because the services provided by the professional are for the benefit of the patient, and the economic retributions are for the benefit of the Institution.

Jorge Iturraspe, with the "Theory of Lending Responsibility", says that the professionals in Health, are not just any "third parties" (They were chosen for their Curriculum, competence test, quality, qualities, scientific knowledge, etc.), the professional apart from having a contract with the institution, has a direct contractual relationship with the patient, and the latter has a reflex relationship (Indirect) with the Institution. When a damage occurs, both are responsible, the Institution responds with the patient and repeats with the professional.

By origin
It is divided into subjective and objective.

The subjective civil liability, is when a predetermined obligation is breached and there must be a guilty conduct; then, to respond one has to be guilty. It is the one that is governed in our legal economy.

The objective civil liability is based on the non-fulfilment that has caused a damage, whether or not it has merited fault, there is still the obligation to repair the damage. Because the result is seen not the conduct of the obligor, even if he had been diligent and prudent.

Obligations of means, of results and of safety in civil liability.

It is of great importance in determining the liability of the Dentist. Non-compliance, which is one of the basic requirements for liability to arise, will depend on the type of obligation.

The obligation of means.

It is the obligation to use all available means for the benefit of the patient's health.

It is in this obligation that we find ourselves, since we have the obligation to put our skills, abilities and knowledge to work in providing our services.

Or, as Ocampo mentions, this obligation includes the following points: Means themselves, Diligence and Circumstances **(OCAMPO CASTELÚ, JORGE. "Diploma of Civil and Criminal Liability of the Doctor" Postgraduate Law- UMSA- 2008).**

Means, according to the complexity of the case (Risks), in a healthy child, in a child with heart disease or other illness. Where and how the child will be attended.

Diligence, celerity, quick attention, but following the protocols for each

29

case (Manual of Oral Health Standards of the Ministry of Health, or other).

Circumstances, cultural situations, customs.

The OBLIGATION OF MEANS, enters in the field of the assistance Odontology, where the patient presents with a visible problem of oral health, is not healthy, something is producing instability, is altering and our commitment is to remedy that problem, and perhaps other problems that arise in the oral examination.

Here, we are required to put our knowledge and experience, with diligence, prudence and expertise to overcome that problem.

We cannot, nor should we, assure the patient of the outcome, much less give guarantees.

The obligation of means is difficult to prove, since it has to be shown that the non-performance does not depend only on the failure to achieve the result, but that it would have to be shown that it could have been possible to achieve it.

The obligation of results.

It is the obligation to heal.
The patient is apparently healthy and wants to solve some defect, something unsightly and the professional is confident of achieving it, is certain of achieving it, is offering a satisfactory result.
This relationship is known as a **contract of performance,** because the professional guarantees the exact fulfilment of an obligation.

It refers to committing to a treatment with an optimal result, and this is how you should do it.

It occurs in Aesthetic Dentistry, Orthodontics, Implants, and others.

Although, some jurists consider that all the specialties of Dentistry should be an obligation of means, because no organism is the same as another and no one reacts the same.

We must remember that the complementary examinations must be attached to the Clinical History, to assume defense if something unforeseen should occur; in the same way, the patient's consent must be obtained, prior truthful, clear and precise information. Without forgetting to note the protocols of care that is being used for each situation (WHO, ICD-10, etc.), by not complying with these protocols we are performing an illegal act, for non-compliance with our rules.

Security obligation

Or mixed, it was created by French doctrine and jurisprudence.

It is more for Medicine, but it is suitable for Buccomaxillofacial Surgery, also for Implantology and others that require hospitalization and postoperative control.

These are the obligations that emanate from public and private health care centers, which assume the obligation of **means** to procure the recovery of health, and the obligation of **results** that the patient will not acquire new diseases or suffer accidents derived from his hospitalization, which is known as nosocomial pathology. (**OCAMPO CASTELÚ, JORGE. "Diploma of Civil and Criminal Liability of the Physician" Postgraduate Law- UMSA- 2008).**

2.1.5. - LEGAL GROUNDS

The Political Constitution of the Bolivian State and the Positive Law protect life, Health and Physical Integrity (Art. 15) as original goods of man, the infraction to this normative supposes the Crime of Injuries or Homicide.

The person criminally responsible for this affectation to health and bodily integrity is also civilly responsible and is obliged to repair the material, corporal and moral damages.

2.   Í.5.Í.- POLITICAL CONSTITUTION OF THE STATE

Article 39.- I. The State shall guarantee the public health service and recognize the private health service; it shall regulate and monitor quality care through sustainable **medical audits** that evaluate the work of its personnel, infrastructure and equipment in accordance with the law.

II. **Negligent** acts or omissions in the exercise of medical practice shall be punishable by law.

2.   Í.5.2. - BOLIVIAN CIVIL CODE

Art. 29Í.- CC (Duty to perform and obligee's right). I. The obligor has the duty to provide exact performance of the due performance. **II.** The obligee, in case of non-performance, can demand performance by the means provided by law.

Article 344.- (REIMBURSEMENT OF DAMAGE). Compensation for damage, by reason of non-performance or delay, includes the loss suffered by the obligee and the gain for which he has been provided, in accordance with the legal provisions.

Article 994.- (REMEDIES). I. The injured party may request, when possible, the compensation of the damage in kind. In adverse case, the compensation shall be assessed by evaluating both the loss suffered by the victim and the lack of profit insofar as it is a direct consequence of the harmful event - emergent damage and loss of profit-. The moral damage must be compensated only in the cases foreseen by the law. **II.-** The judge can equitably reduce the amount of the compensation when fixing it, considering the patrimonial situation of the responsible person who has not acted with malice.

2.2. - ASSESSMENT OF THE ELEMENTS OF CIVIL LIABILITY

2.2.1. - GENERALITIES

It is important to know if the action of the dentist produced the undesired result, or if it occurred despite the presence of the professional in the act without having been the one who originated it.

Mora, proposes the most constant variables that are presented to assess the action of the professional and these are: **(MORA IZQUIERDO, Ricardo. "La responsabilidad del Médico Tratante según el Daño Ocasionando". Manual of the Institute of Legal Medicine. Colombia. 2000)**.

1. Iatrogenic
2. Accident
3. Complication
4. Type of practice
5. Missing Dental

2.2.I.I. - IATROGENSA

It is defined as "Any alteration of the patient's condition produced by the professional". But, in common parlance, the term relates to unavoidable pathological conditions that occur despite the exercise of the profession

33

according to the rules of Lex Artis, Law of Art.

It is an unavoidable, constant damage, which occurs in good professional practice, with an existing causal link, at a time of immediate or early onset and produced by a competent dentist.

For Vargas Alvarado, "The iatrogenic comes to constitute the margin of reliability because it is not required to be infallible, only to be trained to practice their profession" and explains that there are a variety of iatrogenic and these can be: Iatrogenic by diagnostic methods, Iatrogenic by medicines, Iatrogenic by biological products, etc. **(VARGAS ALVARADO E. "Medicina Legal y Forense". (2nd edition) Ed. Trillas. Mexico D.F. 1999.**

2.2.1.2. - ACCIDENT

"*Eventual occurrence that alters the order of things* "[6]. They can be of two types. An accident with an external cause, produced by nature, etc. and another of internal cause, produced by the same professional, which produces an unforeseen damage, which happens suddenly, therefore inevitable, inconstant, with a positive causal link, occurring within a good professional practice in which a competent dentist acted, which usually occurs at a time of immediate onset - when the professional was preparing for the exodontia of a radicular remnant with the elevator, and when the assistant bumped into the surgeon, the latter pushed the elevator into the tissues, causing a serious injury to the tongue. Or different circumstances with the same effects using laser beams, etc.

2.2.1.3. - COMPLICATION

"*Concurrence or meeting of different things, in a negative sense*". Here the damage is inconstant, sometimes foreseeable, it can also be avoidable, the causal link is indirect, the time of occurrence is variable, it occurs within a good professional practice in which a competent dentist acted - the root debris pushed into the maxillary sinus.

2.2.1.4. - TYPE OF PRACTICE

Refers to what type of practice was performed on the patient: Good, bad, malicious or negligent.

GOOD PRACTICE, that the dentist used Lex artis ad-hoc correctly, which nevertheless caused harm.

BAD PRACTICE, See Ch. IX

DOLIOUS PRACTICE, when it damages the volitive and intellectual element when performing a dental performance, when performing orthodontics without having taken any postgraduate course, or when performing general anesthesia on children in the office in violation of the regulations in this regard, or the dental technician who performs the illegal exercise of the profession, placing prostheses or performing exodontia in his laboratory.

GUILTY PRACTICE, when the dentist does not foresee the foreseeable damage or when, having foreseen it, he/she trusts to be able to avoid it without achieving it.

2.2.I.5.   - DENTAL FAULT

It is important to differentiate it from **dental error,** "to be declared civilly liable it is necessary that the act could have been avoided or that the result would have been inexcusable if it had been committed. Therefore, the **fault** is a defect in the act, and the **error** is related to the understanding, with a mistaken concept or a false judgment, a mistake of good faith; then, the liability is in the fault and not in the error. (**COSTAS ARDUZ,**

35

Rolando, COSTAS B. Darío. "Medical Legal Terms in the Bolivian Legislation".2005).

Medicine and dentistry are neither exact nor risk-free sciences, so professionals are subject to the possibility of failure.

2.2.2. - ASSESSMENT OF THE DENTIST'S COMPETENCE

This is a very important issue, because it is about defining the suitability of the treating dentist, to clarify whether he/she was professionally prepared to perform the procedure he/she performed. If he/she was authorized to practice the profession - registered in the Ministry of Health, in the College of Dentists, postgraduate studies, etc.

Their professional competence will be investigated in order to analyze the causes that led to the damage caused by their actions, studying their academic preparation and professional experience.

Judging professional competence is a difficult matter, but we will take some variables recommended by Mora, such as:

Prestige of the university, the state universities are the ones that enjoy prestige. And this is given to them by the graduates, the quality of the teachers, the Research Institutes, when they have one. Private universities, although there are more and more of them every day, the oldest ones are the ones that are fulfilling their objectives every day.

Professional experience, practice differentiates one dentist from another; that is to say, a recent graduate is not the same as another with ten years of practice, a general dentist is not the same as a specialized dentist, a general dentist may have more experience in various specialties than a dentist specialized in only one, but what we need is *where* he practiced, who

36

practiced more and for how long, this differentiates one professional from another, it can be demonstrated with x-rays, medical records, etc.

Postgraduate courses, it is assumed that a professional who has completed postgraduate courses is more competent in that particular field, than another who has not done so, also here we have to note whether it made in a domestic or foreign institution, the prestige of the same, the quality of teachers, and the number of hours of theory and practice, that if it is important. Also that professional with a postgraduate degree is only authorized to perform that specialization and not another, trying to make colleagues understand that it is time to practice only one knowledge and do it well, it is a "commitment to devote himself to a single specialty.

In order to explain the damage, it may be important what kind of technique or practice the university teaches, whether it is:
- Interventionist,
- more clinical,
- more surgical.
- It respects the biological evolution of the organism in the face of the procedures.

- Faster and sacrifices, for the sake of speed, the biological rhythms of each patient.
- It can be considered a mitigating factor. It has to be stolen.
  (CAMPOS, MARIA DE LOURDES B. "Aspectos Clínicos De La Mala praxis En Odontología", 2000.

Teaching experience, the one who teaches his experiences, his knowledge, researches resulting from his work, is the most competent in that specific area, since he studied a lot to achieve that merit. The exceptions would be the teaching obtained by political and partisan influences, very close

37

friendships, or the one who teaches different professorships.

Scientific publications, the dentist who publishes his research, his scientific production is the one who has more knowledge on that subject, than the one who does not. The College of Dentists has a score for publications, whether articles or books, it is an incentive to research or write.

Honorable mentions and awards received, is another criterion for assessing their professional competence.

Refresher courses, the one who participates periodically, either as a speaker or as a student, much more, if he/she exposes what he/she researches.

Curriculum Vitae, serves to assess professional competence, provided they are original and legally acquired.
Subscription to scientific journals, **and** that you are dedicated to reading them and updating your knowledge, will improve your professional competence score.

Number of private patients, this is the point that in my opinion deserves more attention, since satisfied patients bring more patients. In private practice this is what qualifies the competence of the dental professional, the quality of care, and the type of treatment that recommends a competent professional. It should also be taken into account whether attendance at certain dental care is not influenced by low costs.

2.2.3. - ASSESSMENT OF THE DENTIST'S INCOMPETENCE

The damage occurs when the dentist is not professionally competent.

TYPES OF INCOMPETENCE

Vargas Alvarado, distinguishes them by: **(VARGAS ALVARADO E. Medicina Legal y Forense. 2nd Edition. Ed. Trillas. Mexico. D.F. 1999).**

- Disease
- Out of ignorance
- For dishonesty
- Mixed

3.3.1. - Incompetence due to illness, whether physical or mental.

If it is **physical,** it is dramatic for the professional, because it becomes his only means of livelihood and to exercise the profession requires a good physical condition to ensure the suitability of the professional.

If he is **mental, he** may go unnoticed for some time, until he commits some act that denounces his state; or commits dishonest abuses, attempted rape, for example, by placing too much anesthesia that clouds the patient's conscience.

Mora, cites the very old professional who has lost manual or visual ability, who due to incompetence or negligence causes harm to the patient; we cite the dentist who worked for years in a province, who lost his hearing acuity, and did not listen to the complaints of the patients. And he was the only professional in town. **(MORA**

IZQUIERDO, Ricardo. "La responsabilidad del Médico Tratante según el Daño Ocasionando". Manual of the Institute of Legal Medicine. Colombia. 2000).

2.2.3.2. - Incompetence through ignorance

It could be due to a deficient university preparation, lack of updating, or to incur in fields foreign to their specialty. Some cases were seen when the university student is more dedicated to politics, and by means of this he indirectly pressures his teachers to obtain the approval of the subjects or they collaborate because they belong to the same party. These university students, when they graduate by the same means, manage to become "Teachers" in some universities. Then, two types of damage are produced: direct and indirect. **Direct** when they practice the profession and **indirect** when they teach. Another example is the dentist who has recently graduated or is still a student, who sets up his or her practice without having completed the Compulsory Rural Social Service or postgraduate studies and does not have the knowledge or practice necessary to practice.

2.2.3.3. - Incompetence due to dishonesty

The most difficult to control, because it prevails the desire to get money without seeing the consequences, -performing unnecessary endodontics, operations on healthy teeth, or subjecting children to the risks of general anesthesia, to receive more fees-.

2.2.3.4. - Mixed incompetence, the combination of the above manners

2.2.4. - ASSESSMENT OF THE EXISTENCE OF DAMAGE3

This point serves us to note that the harmful act has different forms, which are:

2.2.4. L- CONSTANCY IN THE PRESENTATION OF THE DAMAGE

CONSTANT DAMAGE refers to the presence of damage in the same cases with the same treatment, same diagnosis, same therapy -an antibiogram is recommended before administering antibiotics-, but, we ignore it and administer the medicine that in similar situations gave us good results, we do not follow the protocol for this type of situations. It is a damage that is frequently done.

INCONSTANT or occasional **damage**. Fracture of the maxilla, buccosinusal communication are not frequent.

FORESEEABILITY OF DAMAGE

A distinction must be made between two types of damage:

PREVISIBLE DAMAGE, is the damage that is expected to occur or that could occur - in the exodontia of third molars, especially lower ones, we know that they can fracture if we do not take our precautions.

IMPREVISIBLE DAMAGE, the possibility of the implant migrating into the maxillary sinus is not contemplated.

2.2.4.2. - AVOIDABILITY OF DAMAGE

AVOIDABLE HARM, that which has the opportunity to be avoided - postoperative infection.

INEVITABLE HARM, there is no way to prevent it from occurring, but you can help to prevent its effects from harming you, - Gingival Hyperplasia by ingestion of Phenytoin (Hydantoin), an anticonvulsant that is also administered for Trigeminal Neuralgia.

2.2.4.3. - TIME OF ONSET OF DAMAGE

There are two concomitant possibilities with the act performed

IMMEDIATE DAMAGE or early, soon after injury - almost all injuries, e.g. hot instruments, tears, lacerations in traumatic exodontia, etc.

LATE DAMAGE, long after the intervention of the dentist - Septicemia, Osteomyelitis-.

2.2.5. - ASSESSMENT OF THE CAUSAL LINK

To relate the injury with the tortfeasor, we accept two theories, the "Adequate cause" and the "Condition sine qua non", everything depends on the case. The first one, promulgated by the German school which in summary says "that one must look for which of the facts is legally apt to produce damage and to be able to attribute the author of that fact". And the second, that it has to be a very specific damage, in order to attribute it to the perpetrator.

2.2.2.5.I. - EVALUATION CRITERIA

For the study of the Nexus of Causality, 7 criteria described by Simonín were used, of which only four were used: *Intensity, Topography, Chronology and Evolution.*

Jaume Bofill Soliguer, carried out a study using the criteria of Sir A. Bradford Hill, plus those of Simonín to determine the causal relationship between the event and the damage to health, and determined the following criteria:

1. Strength of association.
2. Constancia
3. Specificity of effect.
4. Time sequence (chronology)
5. Biological gradient (intensity)
6. Biological plausibility

7. Coherence (evolution)

8. Experimentation.

9. Reasoning by analogy

10. Topography

1. - **The strength of association,** "looks for the relationship between the supposed cause and the effect, by means of the Relative Risk". The higher the value of the relative risk (RR), the greater the strength of association; if the relative risk is lower, the causal relationship may be denied.

In some cases, through studies based on evidence ("evidence-based" medicine), there may be databases that can be used for comparison and a scientific basis can be provided - Inflammatory Fibrous Hyperplasia (Epulis, which is the result of ill-fitting dentures, appears after the fitting of the denture, and if that denture was made by a dentist - causal relationship by force of association - then that dentist will be responsible for the treatment.

2. - **Consistency:** "It consists of investigating whether a possible cause-effect relationship has been confirmed by more than one study, in different populations and circumstances by different authors". If so, this criterion is of great value. E.g. FS Paste or Endomethasone (Cause) that were withdrawn from the market due to adverse effects (Effects) on the treated teeth and on the patient's health.

3. - **Specificity of effect:** "If the proposed effect is specifically related to the cause, it is easier to study than if we attribute multiple effects to a single cause". Study the result to find the cause. - Extrusive luxation of the central incisors caused by the excessive force of a fixed orthodontic appliance in an 8 year old girl. Causality, if that piece received a certain treatment with

43

a certain professional, and at a certain time. This helps us to rule out trauma.

4. - **Biological gradient:** (Intensity), "it is a question of evaluating the dose-response curve". The relationship between exodontia and post-exodontic alveolitis or osteitis.

5.   - **Biological plausibility:** This characteristic is limited by the scientific knowledge available at the time of the study. The presence of oral cancer in the oral cavity, HIV.

6. - **Coherence:** (Evolution). The interpretation of causes and effects cannot contradict the behaviour of the disease or injury itself.

7. - **Experimentation:** It is clear that the ability to experimentally reproduce the cause-effect association, or to impact the cause to alter the effect when another mode of experimentation is not possible or **not considered ethical**, help to confirm the causal relationship.

8. - **Reasoning by analogy:** This involves identifying causal associations of a similar nature - accepting the possibility of induction of nephropathy or ototoxicity of a new aminoglycoside antibiotic based on the experience that the rest of the antibiotics in that group produce both lesions.

9. - **Topography,** the relationship between the tortfeasor, the injury and the location of the same, i.e. when a person performs a treatment in a **sector or a field** that does not correspond to it, e.g. intrusion. The Doctor who performs exodontia, the General Dentist who performs Orthodontics, Endodontics, etc. (**ALEJANDRA AGUAD. "Civil Law". School of Law Diego Portales University**).

2.2.5.2.   - ASSESSMENT OF GUILT

This is the basis of civil liability.

In Roman law, a person's conduct was compared to the conduct of a father of a family (pater familia). It was supposed to be the model of prudent and careful behavior. If someone had acted below that conduct, it was a faulty act, while if someone had acted at the same level, it was an act recognized as prudent, diligent and valid. **ROCA FRANCES. "Seminar on the Valuation of Bodily Injury". Bar Association. La Paz - Bolivia. 2007)**

What has to be assessed in this element is the degree of prudence, expertise and diligence that the tortfeasor has had, as Pothier says, quoted by Romero, it has to be assessed the fault **in concreto and in abstracto,** "taking into account that the tortfeasor has not acted to cause the damage; but, if he had conducted himself prudently and diligently, the damage would not have occurred. In order to assess fault **in concreto,** the conscience of the tortfeasor must be examined. **(FRANCO, Manual of Legal and Forensic Medicine, Colombia).**

In order to assess fault **in abstracto,** the conduct of the tortfeasor must be compared with an abstract model, from which the existence or lack of fault can be deduced".

This form of comparison can be made, not with a parent but with the conduct of a good professional, studious, scrupulous, comparing it with the actions of the tortfeasor to determine fault in the latter.

Perhaps in the following case, we can apply the above, analyzing the performance of the dentist and the treatment used.

A 17 year old patient, in good oral health, with healthy and complete

45

dentition, suffered a trauma in the medial anterosuperior region with a root fracture in the apical third of tooth 21 and avulsion of tooth 31.

In the upper jaw, the dentist, without x-rays, tried a kind of splinting with brackets, bands and archwires from 15 to 25 and reinforced with light-curing resins on 21, 22 and 1 1.
In the lower jaw, in the empty socket of 31, he placed an immediate dental implant, without the appropriate recommendations.

At four months, the patient presents apical fistula in 21, mobility and pain in 11 and 22, as well as 41 and 32.

The radiograph shows the very wide fracture line of 21, apical and lateral periodontal thickening in the affected teeth. In the lower jaw, absence of the implant, the radiograph shows marked radiolucency affecting the alveolar wall of the neighbouring teeth - 41 and 32 - and notable periodontal thickening in all the neighbouring teeth.

Each one of us can place ourselves in the dentist's situation and analyze the treatment; whether it was adequate or not, and whether or not the treating professional was at fault, and if so, what element of fault can be attributed to the professional and what type of sanction would correspond to him or her. Of course, the last part is up to the judge.

2.2.5.3. - DIVISION OF BLAME

The most exact division of guilt is conscious guilt and unconscious guilt, which Carrara calls guilt with foresight and guilt without foresight; and which the Romans called "guilt ex ignorancia" and "guilt ex lascivia".

In conscious guilt, the tortfeasor represents the consequences that his act may produce; whereas in unconscious guilt, the agent lacks this

46

representation.

2.2.5.4. - DEGREES OF GUILT

There are three degrees of guilt;
- **Slightest fault**
- **Slight Fault**
- **Serious or gross negligence** (which is equivalent to malice in criminal law).

Culpable breach in **contractual** matters is presumed, in addition to being liable for **slight** negligence. In the **non-contractual** negligent breach, you have to prove that you did not incur in **any act** of negligence, inexperience, recklessness, and demonstrate that you complied with the requirements of the rule.

Some jurists mention that in contractual matters should be liable for slight and gross negligence, and in non-contractual matters for very slight negligence. And, other jurists are of the opinion that in non-contractual matters, there are no degrees of fault.

The slightest fault, our Code does not have a definition in this regard, so we turn to the Colombian Civil Code for a definition, which is expressed in art. 63 "Consists in handling the business of others with that care that even negligent persons or with little prudence, usually use in their own business".

In other words, it is a fact that only extraordinary diligence could have foreseen.

Slight negligence is defined as "lack of diligence and care".

Or is it a fact that only diligent men would have foreseen?

Grave guilt is a fact that all men would have foreseen.

CONCLUSIONS AND RECOMMENDATIONS

CONCLUSIONS

Considering that health professionals have a fundamental training to care for, protect life as a maximum legal good and promote the health of people through the acts of health service in the area or specialty that corresponds to him, and if in this act of the service of patient care is produced some malpractice and cause some iatrogenic either by action or omission and although our legal regulations establish an unlawful consequence with punitive sanction, and it should be clear that the professional undoubtedly does not act with an unlawful conduct of the fraudulent wrongdoing that can be for a reckless conduct or wrongful misconduct which can be treated in the civil area or civil process in which you can seek a conciliatory or reparative way out for the damage suffered.

As we have been able to see in the development of the objectives of this work, in the action of the exercise of the dental profession, there are multiple factors to consider in a dental practice, when it comes to conflicts between professional patient, for an alleged dental malpractice in which it will have to resort to audits and expertise for the clarification of the truth. But above all, an adequate clinical history must be elaborated, and a good informed and signed consent, with all the protocols and observing the procedural, legal and moral ethical regulations.

RECOMMENDATIONS

> To make dentists aware that dentistry is a regulated profession, subject to rules, with precepts that they are obliged to comply with.

> Let the professional know that ignorance of the law is no excuse.

> Recommend that he should take a closer look at the duties that the legal norm imposes on him, and tell him that the harmful result of his actions as a consequence of the violation of the Law does not count on solidarity.

> Solidarity implies, "that each and every one of the intervening agents are individually responsible for the totality of the damage caused".

> That institutions should be instructed when hiring dentists, that they have to demand expertise, experience, skills and abilities not only knowledge, competency tests should be more practical, since the practice provides quality to the dental professional, investigate the veracity of the documents.

> That the institutions in charge of professional practice should ensure that dentists take theoretical and practical examinations on a regular basis.

> That the updating must be constant and permanent.

> Require every dental professional to engage in research, creating a Scientific Committee, seeking some form of funding for such research and perhaps incentive awards.

> That the organizers of refresher courses, seminars, congresses, should know that the non-attendance to these courses is often due

to the high costs and the incompatibility of schedules.

> Like the public, the private practice should have a stricter control, not only of the office but also of the professional.

> Establish a more specific Guide for our profession, or a Protocol
of

Performance or conduct, performed by Dentists.

> Greater participation of the Colleges in public and private institutions, demanding quality control in supplies, instruments and equipment. At the same time, they should demand that dentists participate in dental audits.

> In addition, demand not only quantity in patient care, but quality.

> Dental Colleges should create a Legal Department, with regular updates in this field.

> And, finally, to design projects for Civil Liability **Insurance** for Dentists.

THE MEDICAL HISTORY

As a very relevant recommendation, we emphasize the elaboration of:

The Clinical History is the main evidentiary document in liability lawsuits. Usually its incorporation to the file is the first gesture of the Judge when he takes contact with the written claim **(RODRÍGUEZ, GRILLE, MEDEROS. "Derecho Medico".**
(29) LORENZETTI, R., Responsabilidad Civil De Los Médicos.

In dental medical records, the dentist does an interrogation, makes a good analysis of his patient but does not record this clinicopathological condition in the medical record; he wastes the opportunity to use a document of proof.

Its value as a means of proof lies in the fact that it was made for essentially welfare purposes and, in general, well in advance of the case coming to court.

On the other hand, the fact that it is a document drawn up by one of the parties - the dentist - gives it, for some authors, the character of an "anticipated and written confession" (**Lorenzetti).**

It has been said that what is not recorded in the history is equivalent to what has not been done. More precisely, it can be argued that "what is not recorded in the medical record is presumed not to have been carried out by the dentist, although the contrary can be proved by other means, which in fact is often difficult".

From all of the above we can see the importance of a correct clinical history as part of the professional act.

In particular, when the patient refuses the performance of certain diagnostic or therapeutic means indicated by the dentist, the latter must prove this with documents kept in the medical records, in order to safeguard his liability.

It must be complete, include preoperative, operative and postoperative x-rays, do not forget the general history of the patient, the name of the professional to whom he was referred, the complementary tests, etc., the blood pressure must head this Medical History, the previous state of the patient must also be described, the date and the TIME, everything that the sheet can hold and more. At some point it may be exculpatory or at least a mitigating factor of responsibility.

The PREVIOUS STATUS is important because it indicates "the set of predispositions, of constitutional or acquired anomalies that a subject presents before a determined event" (Daligand et al., 1988), 1988), what type of treatment that tooth already had, if it had some type of infection, if that bone was healthy before serving as a support for a prosthesis or an implant, or if that dental mobility had already been checked, as well as the diastema between the lateral and the canine, if the internal dentine reabsorption was what produced the communication and not the Endodontist's manoeuvre.

At what TIME you received care, it is also important to note to see if you were able to acquire the indicated medications. The dosage is of utmost importance, the route of administration, verify if you complied with the recommendations, rest, diet, etc.

The Dental Medical History is a document that can be used as a means of proof if it is complete and as evidence if it is not.

And, something that is important, if not recorded everything mentioned, you must be very careful to record it later. It is not difficult for a Dental Auditor or handwriting expert to determine which annotations are old and which are not, and a lawsuit for Injuries can be extended to Falsification of a Private Document, typified in Art. 201 Penal Code.

INFORMED AND SIGNED CONSENT

There is an obligation to inform the patient or, where appropriate, the patient's relatives, of the diagnosis of the illness or injury, of the prognosis that can normally be expected from the treatment, of the risks that may arise from the treatment, especially if it is surgical, and, finally, and in the event that the means available in the place where the treatment is applied may be insufficient.

This circumstance should be stated, so that if possible, the patient or his relatives can opt for treatment in another more suitable clinic. (www.negiigencias.medicas.)

It is advisable to explain in simple terms, what treatment you will receive and the chances of success, and if you have understood that this treatment may fail, and despite knowing that you agree to do it, it is advisable to fill out the consent form, which is specific for each patient, and do not forget to sign. If the patient is a minor, the parents or guardians will do it, or the closest relatives if it is extremely urgent. But, never the minor him/herself, no matter how responsible he/she may seem.

It's another disclaimer that at the right time can be a relief.

But, I must mention that in the New Health Law we have to take into account that this consent, comes to constitute a kind of Contract or Agreement between parties (Sandra Kuncar), because it meets all the elements of a contract of Health Services, and with this new model, it does not need to be signed, only to be verbal, and only requires proof of the performance of an odontological act (the wound of exodontia, the needle stick, etc).

OTHER DOCUMENTS

It may be the **prescriptions.** There are individuals who voluntarily hide them, claiming that they were not prescribed the medication or that nothing was recommended. They wait until the problem is exacerbated and it is only then that they come forward demanding reparation, compensation. And, it may happen that in a hurry we have forgotten to write down in the medical history the medications and recommendations to the patient.

With experience in the field, it is preferable to make **prescriptions with a**

54

copy, like invoices, where the patient's name and diagnosis are included. On the reverse side can be printed the recommendations according to the treatment performed, the instructions for Endodontics will not be the same as for a Minor Surgery.

It is very practical this type of prescription with copy especially for injectables, because they are already printed the well-known PREVIOUS TEST for cases of allergy to the medicine that the patient has and does not know it. It can be made as indicated in our Statute in two sheets, one for the pharmacy and another with the indications, but with copy.

Other release documents are **lab tests,** including copies of **orders to dental labs,** and dental labs should keep these orders. Also, orders for transfers, etc. Nor should we forget that prescriptions, lab orders, or any document that is given to the patient, becomes proof of the agreement or contract between the parties.

PROPOSAL

- Malpractice exists in all professions so this issue should be taken into account as a curricular subject in all careers.

- Reform the academic curricular teaching in ethics and morals, for teaching with quality and warmth of the new professionals.

- Greater participation and oversight of professional practice by professional associations and State institutions.

BIBLIOGRAPHY

ROVIERA GOMEZ Rosario. OLMOS SOTO Juan. The Responsibility of the Bolivian Dentist. La Paz - Bolivia. Editorial El Clon. 2009. La Paz - Bolivia. 2009.

MORALES MARTÍNEZ, PEDRO. "The pathologist in the investigation for medical responsibility" Journal of the National Institute of Legal Medicine of Colombia. Volume XVI

IRAOLA, Lidia. Medical-legal liability and malpractice.

MORALES MARTÍNEZ, PEDRO. "The pathologist in the investigation for medical responsibility" Journal of the National Institute of Legal Medicine of Colombia. Volume XVI. Page 85

GISBERT CALABUIG, J.A., "Medicina Legal y Toxicología", Barcelona, Masson-Salvat, 1992.

MORA IZQUIERDO, Ricardo. "La responsabilidad del Médico Tratante según el Daño Ocasionando". Manual of the Institute of Legal Medicine. Colombia. 2000.

VARGAS ALVARADO E. "Medicina Legal y Forense". (2nd edition) Ed. Trillas. Mexico D.F. 1999.

COSTAS ARDUZ, Rolando, COSTAS B. Dario. "Medical Legal Terms in the Bolivian Legislation". 2005.

CAMPOS, MARIA DE LOURDES B. "Clinical Aspects Of Dental Malpractice", 2000.

VARGAS ALVARADO E. Forensic Medicine. 2nd Edition. Ed. Trillas.

56

Mexico. D.F. 1999

JAUME BOFILL SOLIGUER "Qualified Medical Experts", Tarragona-Spain.

ALEJANDRA AGUAD. "Civil Law". Diego Portales University School of Law.

ROCA FRANCES. "Seminar on the Valuation of Bodily Injury". Bar Association. La Paz - Bolivia. 2007

FRANCO, Manual of Legal and Forensic Medicine. Colombia.

COSTA ARDUZ Rolando, COSTA B. Dario. Medical Legal Terms in the Bolivian Legislation. 2005

RODRIGUEZ A. Civil Liability Derived from the Medical Act. Colombia. 2004

VILLARROEL BUSTIOS, CESAR. "Obligations" Law Degree. UMSA. 2005.

LUNA YAÑEZ Alberto. "Obligations". Printing. Artyk productions. 1996

DE BRIGARD PEREZ Ana. Fault in medical liability. Colombia.

SABAT, JOSÉ. "Diploma in Civil and Criminal Liability of Physicians". Argentine Teacher. Law. UMSA.2008

OCAMPO CASTELÚ, JORGE. "Diploma of Civil and Criminal Liability of the Physician" Postgraduate Law- UMSA- 2008.

RODRÍGUEZ, GRILLE, MEDEROS, "Medical Law". LORENZETTI,

R., Responsabilidad Civil De Los Médicos.

POLITICAL CONSTITUTION OF THE STATE (2009). Legal Gazette. 1st. Edition. La Paz- Bolivia.

PENAL CODE LAW NO. 1768 OF 10 MARCH 1997

BOLIVIAN CRIMINAL PROCEDURE CODE

LAW 3131 OF THE PROFESSIONAL PRACTICE

BOLIVIAN CIVIL CODE

MEDICAL JOURNAL LA PAZ. Dr. ROXANA BEMORDET BURGOS PORTILLO.
"Member of the Committee". Editorial Revista Médica del C.M.D.L.P. La Paz - Bolivia. 2014

CODE OF THE COLLEGE OF DENTISTS OF BOLIVIA.

CODE OF THE MEDICAL COLLEGE OF BOLIVIA.

CODE OF ETHICS AND MEDICAL DEONTOLOGY. BOLIVIA.

WEBGRAPHY
www.negligenciasmedicas

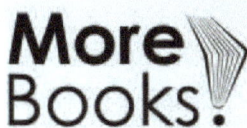
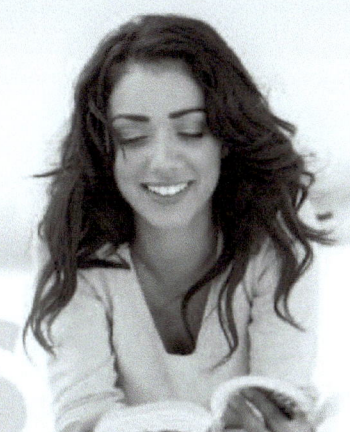
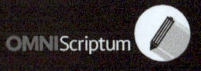

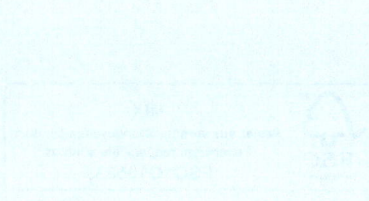

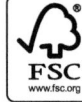
Printed by Books on Demand GmbH, Norderstedt / Germany